All About ARTHRITIS

By Laura Flynn R.N., B.N., M.B.A., in consultation with her nurse educator associates and physicians who assisted in contributing and editing.

ISBN No: 978 1 896616 53 7

© 2010, 2017 Mediscript Communications Inc.

The publisher, Mediscript Communications Inc., acknowledges the financial support of the Government of Canada through the Canadian Book Fund for our publishing activities.

www.mediscript.net

Printed in Canada

Book and Front Cover design by:
Brian Adamson, www.AdamsonGraphics.net

AR1002010

2

ALL ABOUT BOOKS

Trusted • Reliable • Certified

- 40+ titles available
- Comply with accreditation and regulatory bodies
- Suitable for caregivers, boomers with elderly parents, health workers, auxiliary health staff & patients
- Self study style with "test yourself" section
- Health On the Net (HON) certified

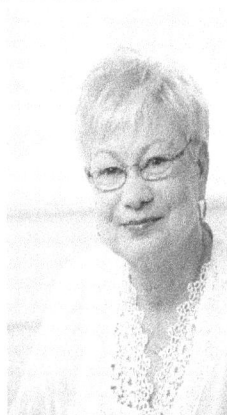

Some of our titles:

Alzheimers Disease	Arthritis	Multiple Sclerosis
Pain	Strokes	Elder Abuse
Falls Prevention	Incontinence	Nutrition & Aging
Personal Care	Positioning	Confusion
Transferring people	Care of the Back	Skin Care

For complete list of titles go to www.mediscript.net

Contact: 1 800 773 5088
Fax 1800 639 3186 • Email; mediscript30@yahoo.ca

CONTENTS

INTRODUCTION

This This book provides basic, non controversial and trusted information that can help a wide spectrum of readers.

The primary objective of the information is to help a person provide effective quality care to a loved one or someone in his or her care.

Your role as a caregiver could mean the older person in your care is a family member or loved one, or you may be a non family member who is helping out a friend. Alternatively, you may be a paid health worker providing quality care for a client. With this in mind, we will alternate between referring to family members, loved ones, older persons and clients.

All the information is reliable and was written by a group of eminent nurse educators who ensured the information complies with best practice guidelines and satisfies the various accreditation and regulatory bodies. Because there is so much unreliable information on the internet, you can be assured the "All About" publications are HON (Health On the Net) certified.

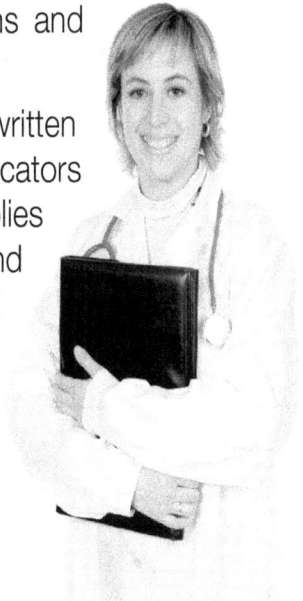

This book can be an invaluable aid to:

- A caregiver caring for a relative or friend;
- A health worker seeking a reference aid;
- A patient or person with arthritis;
- Any person involved in health care wishing to expand his or her knowledge.

SOMETHING TO THINK ABOUT...

Only I can change my life.

No one can do it for me.

Carol Burnett

AN IMPORTANT MESSAGE
FROM THE PUBLISHER

Each person's treatment, advice, medical aids, physical therapy and other approaches to health care are unique and highly dependant upon the diagnosis and overall assessment by the medical team.

We emphasize therefore that the information within this book is not a substitute for the advice and treatment from a health care professional.

This book provides generic information concerning the issues around arthritis and common sense, well-established care practices for caring for someone with this condition.

With all this in mind, the publishers and authors disclaim any responsibility for any adverse effects resulting directly or indirectly from the suggestions contained within this book or from any misunderstanding of the content on the part of the reader.

The teacher of the earth science class was lecturing on map reading.

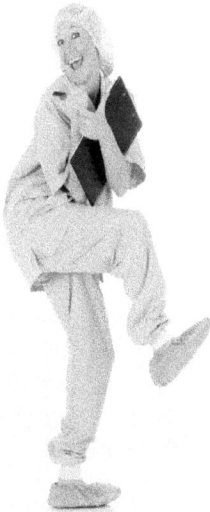

After explaining about latitude, longitude, degrees and minutes, the teacher asked, "Suppose I asked you to meet me for lunch at 23 degrees, 4 minutes north latitude and 45 degrees, 15 minutes east longitude?"

After a confused silence, a voice volunteered:

"I guess you'd be eating alone!"

Source: www.AhaJokes.com

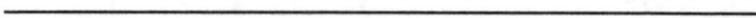

HOW MUCH DO YOU KNOW?

It helps to figure out how much you know before you start. In this way you will have an idea as to the gaps in your knowledge prior to reading the content. Please circle to indicate the best answer. Remember, at this stage, you are not expected to know all the answers:

1. What does the word "arthritis" mean?

a. A bone disease

b. Inflammation of the joint

c. An infectious disease

d. A viral disease

2. Which statement is most true?

a. Only old people get arthritis.

b. There is only one kind of arthritis.

c. The symptoms of arthritis are always the same.

d. People of all ages can have arthritis.

3. What is the best definition for "crepitus"?

a. A grating sound caused by bones rubbing together

b. Swelling, warmth and pain of a joint

c. The point where two bones meet

d. A drug used to treat arthritis

4. What is the common factor in all forms of arthritis?

a. Fever

b. Swelling of the joints

c. Joint and musculoskeletal pain

d. Arthritis starts at the site of a previous injury

5. Which of the following is a risk factor for osteoarthritis (OA)?

a. Age

b. Smoking

c. Viral infection

d. Diet low in calcium

6. At what age do most people with rheumatoid arthritis (RA) develop the disease?

a. Infants to school age

b. 20 to 40

c. 25 to 50

d. 70s and 80s

7. Which statement about RA is most true?

a. It mainly affects joints in the fingers, wrists and knees.

b. Pain occurs with activity and improves with rest.

c. The disease is common in persons who are obese.

d. The disease only affects the joints in the body.

ANSWERS

1. b. The word arthritis means "inflammation of the joint".

2. d. Older people are more likely to have arthritis but it is not just a disease of the old.

3. a. "Crepitus" is a grating sound and sensation caused by bones rubbing together.

4. c. The common factor in all forms of arthritis is joint and musculoskeletal pain.

5. a. Eighty per cent of people over the age of 65 have some degree of osteoarthritis (OA) that can be seen on an X-ray.

6. c. The usual age of onset of rheumatoid arthritis (RA) is 25 to 50, although it can affect people of all ages.

7. a. RA mainly affects joints in the fingers, wrists and knees.

ABOUT ARTHRITIS

As a caregiver, you may know that arthritis causes pain in the joints. But what else do you know about the disease? Many people have false ideas about arthritis. Common fallacies are that:

- There is just one kind of arthritis
- The symptoms of arthritis are always the same
- Only old people get arthritis

Let's look at these beliefs one by one.

Is there just one kind of arthritis?

No. Over 100 conditions fall under the heading of "arthritis". Some forms of arthritis cause only mild distress and may affect just one joint. Others can have a severe effect on the entire body. Some forms of arthritis can result in deformity and disability.

Are the symptoms of arthritis always the same?

Despite what many people believe, the symptoms are not always the same. The disease pattern, the severity of pain and disability, and the site of the symptoms can differ for different forms of arthritis. For example, in gout, one type of arthritis, the main symptom is often sudden, acute pain in the great toe.

Do only old people get arthritis?

Older people are more likely to have arthritis. It is not just a disease of the old, however. Many young adults in the prime of their lives develop arthritis. Some forms of the disease even affect children.

KEY TERMS

Alternative medicine

Treatment methods used in place of conventional medicine

Autoimmune disease

A disease caused by problems with the immune system. The body fails to recognize its own cells and creates antibodies against them.

Complementary medicine

Treatments used to complement (not replace) conventional medicine

Crepitus

A grating sound and sensation caused by bones rubbing together

Glucosamine and chrondoitin

A nutritional supplement that is widely used to treat the symptoms of osteoarthritis

Inflammation

Swelling, warmth and pain of the joint

Nodule

A small, rounded mass

NSAIDs

Non steroidal anti-inflammatory drugs

Remission

A period of time when symptoms of a disease disappear. A remission does not usually last long.

Rheumatoid nodules

Firm, non tender nodules that are most often found in the wrist, knee, elbow, and finger joints

THR

Total hip replacement

TKR

Total knee replacement

WHAT IS ARTHRITIS?

The word arthritis means "inflammation of the joint". Inflammation causes swelling, redness, warmth and pain in the joint(s). Some forms of arthritis do not cause these symptoms. Most forms, however, do cause inflammation of the affected joints as the body attempts to respond to injury. The common factor in all forms of arthritis is joint and musculoskeletal pain.

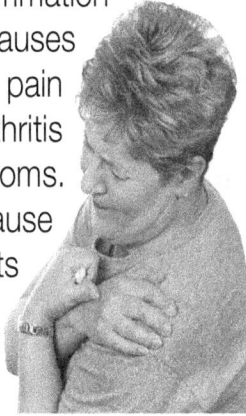

Some types of arthritis occur more often than others. Here we will discuss two of the more common forms of arthritis – osteoarthritis (OA) and rheumatoid arthritis (RA).

HOW JOINTS WORK

Now that you know that arthritis affects the joints, let's look at how the joints work. A joint is any point where two bones meet. There are over 100 joints in the body. Some of these joints move slightly or not at all. Others move freely. Synovial joints are the most complex type of joint. They are found in many parts of the body, including the knees, shoulders, hips, and fingers. Synovial joints consist of:

- **Cartilage:** a smooth surface that cushions the end of the bones and acts as a shock absorber

- **Joint capsule:** a membrane sac that encloses the joint space and retains fluid

- **Joint space or joint cavity:** a space between the ends of the two bones that contains synovial fluid

- **Synovium:** an inner lining inside the joint capsule which produces synovial fluid

- **Synovial fluid:** a fluid that nourishes the joint and keeps it moist

- **Ligaments, tendons, and muscles:** tissues that allow the joint to move and that help keep the bones stable. Ligaments attach one bone to another. Tendons connect muscles to bone.

In a healthy joint, all of the parts of the joint work together to reduce friction. The joint capsule holds everything in place and movement occurs without pain.

OSTEOARTHRITIS

Osteoarthritis, or OA, is the most common form of arthritis. This chronic disease affects about 80% of Canadians by the time they reach the age of 75. In the U.S. nearly 21 million people over the age of 45 have OA. It has been estimated that 41 million Americans 65 years and over will have OA by the year 2030.

> ## CONSIDER FOR A MOMENT ...
>
> How many people with
>
> OA do you know?

OA is a non inflammatory disease of the joints that results in a breakdown of cartilage over time. You've already learned that cartilage cushions the end of the bones and acts as a shock absorber. In a healthy person, cartilage breaks down and then restores itself. In the person with OA, cartilage breaks down much faster than it can be repaired. When cartilage is gone, bone surfaces grate together causing pain. Pain is also felt in the muscles and supporting tissues. Bony spurs grow from the bone edges, leading to changes in the shape of the bone and joint, and synovial fluid increases.

WHAT ARE THE RISK FACTORS FOR OA?

The exact cause of OA is not known. Several factors, however, called "risk factors", make it more likely that someone will get OA. These factors include:

Age

80% of people over the age of 65 have some degree of OA that can be seen on an x-ray. As the number of older adults increase, we can expect that OA will become more common over time.

Obesity

Obese persons are at increased risk for OA, mainly OA of the knees. Standing or walking exerts a pressure of up to 6 times a person's body weight on the knees and up to 3 times the body weight on the hips. So you can see why obesity can lead to joint problems.

Genetics

OA is not thought to be a genetic disease, although there is an increased risk for those whose parents had the disease.

Injury or trauma

An example would be an injury caused by lifting over a period of time.

Lack of exercise

Regular exercise lowers the risk of OA in several ways. It helps strengthen supporting muscles, tendons and ligaments, it promotes cartilage growth and it assists in weight control.

CONSIDER FOR A MOMENT ...

Do you have any of these risk factors for OA?

WHAT ARE THE SYMPTOMS OF OA?

OA can be present for many years before symptoms appear. The first symptom of OA is often the slow onset of aching joint pain. OA most often affects joints in the knees, hips, spine, ankles, and hands. Pain often occurs with activity and is relieved by rest. Joint stiffness occurs after periods of inactivity. Stiffness improves as the person moves around.

DIAGNOSING OA

There is no one test for OA. The diagnosis is based upon the following:

History

The history includes the symptoms. There may be local pain and stiffness with little or no swelling. The affected joints are usually weight-bearing ones as well as joints in the spine and in the hand. The pain may occur with activity but improve with rest.

Physical exam

Some joints may be enlarged. Limited range of motion may be present. **Crepitus** is a grating sound and sensation caused by bones rubbing together. It may be heard and felt upon movement of one or more affected joints. Advanced disease may cause some joints to "lock" as the person walks. The disease can also result in bony growths in the hands.

X-ray findings

X-rays may show bony spurs and a narrowed joint space due to wearing away of cartilage.

Lab findings

A lab test can be done to rule out other types of arthritis such as RA and gout.

TREATMENT FOR OA

There is no cure for OA. The disease, however, can be managed. Below are some steps for managing OA:

Weight loss

This is helpful if the person is obese. Excess weight causes stress on weight-bearing joints such as the hips and knees.

Exercise

Exercise allows synovial fluid to warm and thin out. This makes it easier for cartilage in the joint to absorb the fluid. As the cartilage absorbs fluid, it swells and acts as a better cushion against friction. Exercise allows cartilage to do its job. Only through exercise can cartilage get rid of waste products and do the job it is supposed to do. More than one kind of exercise may be helpful. Flexibility exercises help keep the joints

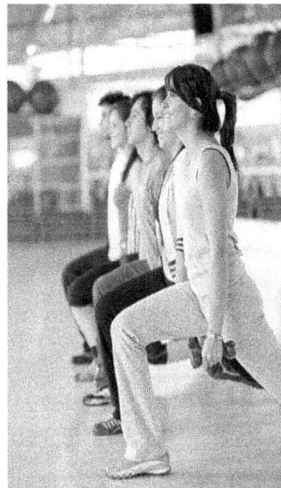

from becoming stiff. Strengthening exercises help maintain or increase strength. Low-impact aerobic exercises such as walking, swimming, water aerobics and stationary biking, have many benefits. Aerobic exercise helps maintain a healthy weight, improve overall fitness, and reduce pain. It also promotes strength and flexibility.

Before starting any exercise program, it is important to consult a physician to ensure the best plan for the person with arthritis.

Medication

- Acetaminophen is often used to treat OA. Tylenol is a common form of acetaminophen. It is used for pain relief but does not reduce inflammation. Acetaminophen should be taken only as directed. Overdosing can result in liver damage.

- Non steroidal anti-inflammatory drugs (NSAIDs) help reduce stiffness, pain and swelling of the joints. Long-term use at high dosages, however, has been linked to possibly serious side effects. These side effects include internal bleeding, high blood pressure and heart and kidney problems. Vioxx, one of the most widely used NSAIDs, was freely withdrawn from the worldwide market by Merck & Co. Inc. in 2004. The decision to withdraw

Vioxx was based upon findings from a drug trial that showed an increased risk of heart attack and stroke after 18 months. People taking NSAIDs should be encouraged to learn about the possible side effects and to report any that are present to their doctor.

- Stronger pain relief meds (e.g. long-acting opoids) are sometimes ordered for severe pain.

- A topical pain reliever works to reduce pain. The cream is rubbed into the skin over a joint. It is often used to help control pain in the knees and hands.

- Steroids are sometimes injected into acutely inflamed joints. The process should be done no more than four times in a one-year period.

Glucosamine and chrondoitin

This is a nutritional supplement that is widely used to treat the symptoms of OA. Further research is needed to find out how well the product works.

Heat or cold therapy

Some people find that applying heat (e.g. hot shower) helps reduce joint pain. Cold treatments to a joint may help decrease the swelling and pain.

Surgery

This is sometimes needed to restore joint motion when the disease has extremely limited joint function. Surgery may involve cleaning or removing damaged tissue or realigning or fusing joints. Fusing involves joining two bones together. Replacement surgery involves removal of part or all of the damaged bone and replacing it with artificial products. Total hip replacement (THR) and total knee replacement (TKR) are two common types of surgery done to restore joint function. If you are caring for a loved one following surgery, such as a THR or TKR, be sure to follow his or her post-op treatment plan.

RHEUMATOID ARTHRITIS

Rheumatoid arthritis (RA) is a chronic, systemic and inflammatory disease and is classified as an autoimmune connective tissue disease. An autoimmune disease is one caused by problems with the immune system. The body fails to recognize its own cells and creates antibodies against them. These new antibodies cause local and systemic reactions.

RA causes inflammation in the joints and joint deformity. The disease is not as common as OA although about 3 million people in the U.S. have it.

In Canada RA affects about 1 of every 100 persons. The disease is more common among women than men (3:1 ratio). By the age of 65, though, men are equally affected. The usual age of onset is 25 to 50, although it can affect people of all ages. It even occurs sometimes in toddlers.

WHAT ARE THE RISK FACTORS FOR RA?

It is believed that more than one factor causes RA. Some, but not all, of the people affected by RA have other family members with the disease. It is possible that bacteria or a virus may trigger the disease, although this has not been definitely proven.

WHAT ARE THE SYMPTOMS OF RA?

RA starts out with increasing fatigue for most affected persons. Other symptoms are widespread musculoskeletal pain, low-grade fever, and decreased appetite. Weight loss occurs. The disease attacks the joint lining (synovium), causing inflammation and damage to cartilage and bone. The joints may also be swollen and range of motion decreased. RA causes pain and stiffness in the joints. Unlike OA, the pain with RA does not go away with rest.

Joint stiffness occurs after periods of inactivity. Morning stiffness may take a long time to resolve. Joints on both sides of the body tend to be affected. For example, if one knee is affected, the other knee will be affected as well. Rheumatoid nodules tend to occur. A nodule is a small, rounded mass. Rheumatoid nodules are firm and non tender. They are most often found in the wrist, knee, elbow, and finger joints. Joint deformities occur over time.

RA is often marked by flare-ups and remissions that sometimes last for many years. Over time, the episodes of inflammation lead to a loss of joint function. The disease is not limited to the joints. RA affects connective tissue anywhere in the body - the heart, lungs, kidneys, eyes, and skin. The joints are mainly affected.

DIAGNOSING RA

Diagnosis stems from the symptoms, the pain pattern, and lab and x-ray results. A lab test to detect the rheumatoid factor (RF) can help to diagnose RA. It may take some time, however, for RF levels to rise in someone affected by RA. As well, RF has been found in persons with no signs of the disease.

TREATMENT FOR RA

Early diagnosis and treatment can help prevent joint damage. Treatment includes meds, rest, an exercise program, protection of the joints and possibly surgery if other treatment measures do not work. The aim is to control pain, maintain movement of the joints, and prevent deformities from occurring. Rest must be balanced with an exercise program.

Did you know that stress tightens muscles and worsens pain? On the other hand, relaxation techniques, such as meditation, listening to music, or deep breathing exercises may help to reduce pain. Heat or cold therapy may also be useful for RA. Different types of meds are used to treat the disease. You should always be aware of potential side effects of any drugs and report these to the physician.

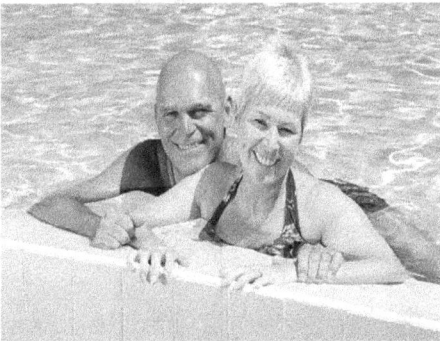

Osteoarthritis	Rheumatoid Arthritis
• The disease involves the breakdown of cartilage over time	• A progressive autoimmune disease that causes inflammation of the lining of the joints
• Usually affects joints on one side of the body	• Usually affects joints on both sides of the body (e.g. both knees, both hips)
• Mainly affects weight-bearing joints (e.g. hips, knees, ankles), spine and joints in the fingers	• Mainly affects joints in the fingers, wrists, and knees
• Common symptoms are local pain and stiffness of the joints although swelling is usually not present	• Common symptoms are joint pain, tenderness, redness, warmth and swelling
• Pain occurs with activity and improves with rest	• Rest does not improve pain. Pain is also common at night.
• Age of onset is generally 40s and 50s	• Usually strikes between the ages of 25 and 50, although it can affect people of all ages.
• The disease does not affect any other systems	• The disease is systemic and may affect the lungs, heart, and skin
• Common in persons who are obese	• Affected persons are usually of average to below average weight for their size
	(Black, Hawks, & Keene, 2001)

CARE CONSIDERATIONS

Now that you know more about arthritis, what can you do to assist people with OA and RA?

Where possible, encourage your loved one to take an active role in managing the disease.

Caregivers and their families should learn about arthritis, find out what works best for chronic pain, and take part in the treatment program. An arthritis self-management program is offered in most parts of Canada. This is a six-week self-help program. It gives people with arthritis a chance to learn more about the disease and also to meet others in the same situation. If you wish to find out about programs in your area you may phone the Arthritis Society at 1-800-321-1433. Chapters of the Arthritis Foundation in the U.S. offer similar sessions. The contact number for the Foundation is 1-800-283-7800.

Encourage arthritis sufferers to inform their health care providers about all the treatments they are using.

Arthritis is a chronic disease with no known cure. Despite medical treatment, many people with arthritis have pain, disability, deformity, and decreased quality of life. Many arthritic sufferers have turned to alternative and/or complementary medicine to try and find a cure or to improve the quality of their lives. **Alternative medicine** refers to treatment methods used in place of conventional medicine. Conventional medicine is taught in western medical schools. **Complementary medicine** is used to complement (not replace) conventional medicine.

Various types of alternative and complementary treatments are in common use today. Three examples are herbal medicine, acupuncture and reflexology. Herbal medicine is the use of certain herbs for their medicinal effects. Acupuncture is a traditional Chinese treatment used to decrease pain, control nausea and aid relaxation. It involves the use of thin needles to apply pressure to certain points of the body. Reflexology is a way of treating certain conditions by massaging the soles of the feet or the palms of the hands. It follows principles similar to acupuncture.

Side effects sometimes occur from mixing treatments (e.g. medicinal herbs and prescribed and over-the-counter drugs). It's important for people to inform their health care providers about all the treatment methods they are using.

Don't ignore pain.

Chronic pain can be a serious challenge for many persons with arthritis. Chronic pain can be mentally and physically exhausting. Advise your loved one to take meds as directed and to rest joints that are painful and swollen. Remind him that stress may increase muscle tension and worsen any pain. Relaxation techniques may help to reduce anxiety. Some people find massage therapy helpful. Others listen to music, practice deep breathing exercises or meditation.

Remember that it's important to balance activity and rest.

Chronic pain can be very tiring. Tell your loved one that it's okay to take a short rest period if she's tired. It is also important to get enough sleep at night.

Assist with activities of daily living.

As the disease progresses, your family member may have trouble doing simple activities. Dressing may pose a problem. He may need to change the type of clothing he usually wears. Velcro fasteners, rather than buttons or zippers, will make it easier for a person with pain or limited hand movement to dress alone. Large-handled eating utensils, raised toilet seats, and higher chairs are examples of how equipment can be adapted to assist with daily living. Canes or walkers may help the person with walking. Joint problems make falls more likely. Ensure a clear path for walking. A number of health care professionals (e.g. an occupational therapist or a physiotherapist) can be quite helpful in suggesting changes to meet the needs of people with arthritis.

Observe and report signs of depression.

Chronic pain, disability and deformity may lead to feelings of depression that may require medical help. The depressed person may look sad and cry often. Other common signs are feelings of despair, lack of energy, changes in appetite, disturbed sleep pattern, and decreased sexual interest. If your family member is depressed, tell the health care professional. Take threats of suicide seriously. Notify the appropriate person right away.

Assist with any other aspects of the treatment plan.

Exercise or diet may be a part of the person's daily routine. Perhaps he is recovering from surgery such as a THR or a TKR. In any case, always follow the treatment plan. Ask questions if you are not sure about any aspect of care. Report any unusual or surprising findings to the health care professional.

CASE EXAMPLE

You have been assigned to care for a 75-year-old man in his own home. Bill has osteoarthritis (OA). The disease has affected the joints of his hands so that he requires help with activities of daily living. He uses a cane to assist with walking.

Bill tries to do as much as he can for himself during the day. He dresses himself in the morning but has trouble doing so. He often becomes tired in the afternoons but refuses to "give in" to his illness by resting.

Several of Bill's friends also have OA. One of these friends recently told him about a new herb that "does wonders" for improving the symptoms of OA. Bill tells you that he is going to get some of that herb too. You know that he also takes meds prescribed by a physician.

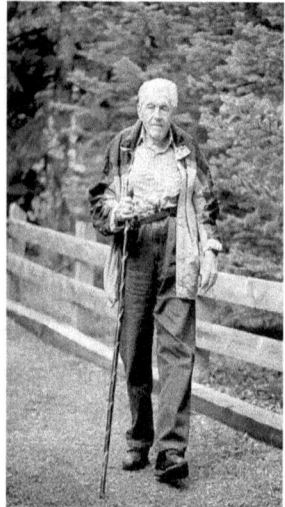

From the information given above, can you identify four key issues (possible concerns) related to Bill's care. *How could you help with each of these issues?*

YOUR ANSWERS TO CASE EXAMPLE

SUGGESTED ANSWERS TO CASE EXAMPLE

The column on the left identifies four key issues outlined in the case example. The column on the right indicates how you can assist with each issue.

Key Issue	How You Can Help
• Use of a cane	• Ensure a clear pathway to prevent falls.
• Has trouble dressing himself	• Inquire about the use of clothing (e.g. pants with Velcro fasteners in place of buttons) that would make it easier for him to dress himself.
• Tired in the PM but won't rest	• Reassure him that it's okay to take a nap in the PM if he is tired.
• Planning to use herbs. Already on meds prescribed by her physician.	• Encourage him to inform his physician about herbal use to prevent possible side effects from mixing the two treatments.

CONCLUSION

Despite what many people believe, arthritis is not a single disease. It is a broad term that covers over 100 diseases and conditions. Arthritis affects people of all ages but is more common among older adults. With our aging population, we can expect to see many more people with arthritis over time.

There is no cure for arthritis. People need to learn more about this chronic condition. They also need to become actively involved in the management of it. Many volunteer organizations provide information and support to interested persons. Conventional and alternative treatment options are available. The role of the caregiver is to provide information, understanding and support to people with arthritis.

RESOURCES

Below are web sites from various arthritis-related organizations. These web sites provide important information to persons affected by arthritis and/or to professionals involved in their care.

American Pain Foundation (APF)

http://www.painfoundation.org/default.asp

A non-profit organization that provides information and that advocates for clients with pain.

Arthritis Foundation

http://www.arthritis.org

Provides leadership in the prevention, control, and cure of arthritis and related diseases. Also supports arthritis research. Offers a wide number of community-based services to improve the lives of those with arthritis.

Association of Rheumatology Health Professionals (ARHP)

http://www.rheumatology.org/arhp/index.asp

An association of non-physician healthcare professionals focusing on rheumatology.

Johns Hopkins Arthritis Centre

http:www.hopkins-arthritis.org

Provides an educational program for healthcare professionals about diseases that cause arthritis and their treatments.

National Institute of Arthritis and Musculoskeletal and Skin Diseases (NIAMS)

http://www.nih.gov/niams

Leads the federal government's research efforts in arthritis and musculoskeletal and skin diseases.

The Arthritis Society

www.arthritis.ca

Provides different treatment and education programs for people with arthritis.

CONSIDER FOR A MOMENT ...

What arthritis resources are
available for caregivers and families
in the area where you live?

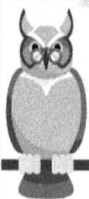

CHECK YOUR KNOWLEDGE

1. What is "arthritis"?

2. How do joints work?

3. How do OA and RA differ?

4. Describe four treatment options for arthritis.

5. How would you care for a client with arthritis?

TEST YOURSELF

Please circle to indicate the best answer:

1. Which of the following indications best describes inflammation of a joint?

a. Enlarged and stiff joint

b. A grating sound in the joint

c. Limited movement in the joint

d. Swelling, redness, warmth and pain in the joint

2. How many people over the age of 45 in the U.S. have OA?

a. Nearly 7 million

b. Nearly 21 million

c. 41 million

d. 210 million

3. How can you lower your risk of OA?

a. Exercise regularly

b. Get lots of sleep at night

c. Begin relaxation classes

d. There is nothing you can do to lower your risk as OA is a genetic disease.

4. Which statement about RA is most true?

a. The pain with RA does not go away with rest.

b. It is common in persons who are obese.

c. It usually affects joints on one side of the body.

d. It mainly affects weight-bearing joints.

5. What is the best description of "alternative medicine"?

a. Another name for conventional medicine

b. Treatment methods that complement conventional medicine

c. Treatment methods used in place of conventional medicine

d. A type of medicine practiced in Japan

6. Which strategy would NOT be helpful for a person with RA who has a painful and swollen joint?

a. Vigorous exercise while the joint is inflamed

b. Rest the joint that is painful and swollen

c. Relaxation techniques to reduce stress

d. Meditation

7. What advice would be most helpful for an obese person with OA who has decided to begin an exercise program?

a. Use weights for the strengthening exercises.

b. Include flexibility and aerobic exercises.

c. Avoid exercise until obesity has been controlled.

d. Consult a physician to ensure the best exercise plan for the person.

ANSWERS

1. **d.** Inflammation causes swelling, redness, warmth and pain in the joint(s).

2. **b.** In the U.S. nearly 21 million people over the age of 45 have OA. It has been estimated that 41 million Americans 65 years and over will have OA by the year 2030.

3. **a.** Regular exercise lowers the risk of OA in several ways. It helps strengthen supporting muscles, tendons and ligaments, it promotes cartilage growth and it assists in weight control.

4. **a.** Unlike OA, the pain with RA does not go away with rest.

5. **c.** "Alternative medicine" refers to treatment methods that are used in place of conventional medicine.

6. **a.** Vigorous exercise is NOT recommended while the joint is inflamed.

7. **d.** Before starting any exercise program, it is important to consult a physician to ensure the best plan for the person with arthritis.

REFERENCES

Anderson, D. (Ed.). (2002). Mosby's medical, nursing, & allied health dictionary (6th ed.). St. Louis, MO: Mosby.

Black, J. M., Hawks, J.H., & Keene, A. M. (2001). Medical-Surgical nursing. (6th ed.). St. Louis, MO: W.B. Saunders.

Lueckenotte, A. (2000). Gerontologic Nursing (2nd ed.). St. Louis: Mosby.

National Center for Chronic Disease Prevention and Health Promotion (CDC) (2005).

Arthritis: Overview. Retrieved May 31st, 2005, http://www.cdc.gov/arthritis/arthritis/index.htm

National Institute of Arthritis and Musculoskeletal and Skin Diseases (NIAMS) (2002).

Handout on health:Osteoarthritis. Retrieved June 21, 2005, http://www.niams.nih.gov/hi/topics/arthritis/oahandout.htm

Roberts, D. (2003). Alternative therapies for arthritis treatment: Part 1. Orthopaedic Nursing, 22 (5), 335-342.

Rooney, J. (2004). Oh, those aching joints: What you need to know about arthritis. Nursing 2005, 34 (11), 58-63.

Saladin, K. (2004). Anatomy and physiology: The unity of form and function. (3rd ed). Boston, MA: McGraw Hill.

Sorrentino, S. (2004). Mosby's Canadian textbook for the support worker. Toronto,ON: Mosby.

The Arthritis Society (2005a). Osteoarthritis. Retrieved May 31st, 2005, from: http://www.arthritis.ca/types%20of%20arthritis/osteoarthritis/default.asp?s=1

The Arthritis Society (2005b). Types of arthritis. Retrieved May 31st, 2005, http://www.arthritis.ca/types%20of%20arthritis/default.asp?s=1

The Arthritis Society (2005c). Arthritis self-management program. Retrieved May 31st,

2005, http://www.arthritis.ca/programs%20and%20resources/arth%20self%20man/default.asp?s=1